In Search of Authenticity
A Meditation On Martial Arts

by
Raymond Towers

Copyright 2006 UKTQF

All rights reserved. No part of this book may be used or reproduced in any manner whatsoever without written permission, except in the case of brief quotations embodied in critical articles or reviews.

Published 2006 by the United Kingdom Taiji Qigong Foundation
ISBN 1-4116-7645-9

First Published by UKTQF 2006
www.uktqf.co.uk

Text copyright 2006 by Raymond Towers
Cover design copyright 2006 Marc Wongsam
Inside illustrations copyright 2006 Glennie Kindred

Contents

In Search of Authenticity	5
Introduction	7
Week One - Week Fifty-Two	13 - 67
Postscript	70
Xingyiquan Classics	72
The Song of Fighting	73
Taijiquan	76
Taiji in Taijiquan	77
Baguazhang	80
The Song of Circle Walking	81

Foreword for

In Search of Authenticity

As the title informs the reader this small book is a meditation, a product of deep thought and reflection, and as such will be of most value to those prepared to approach it in the same spirit of unhurried consideration. We often hear such terms as 'information society' and 'knowledge economy' used as though information and knowledge are interchangeable, but real knowledge only comes with understanding which, in the field of martial arts as in many other areas, comes only with practice. While this book is the result of a lifetime's knowledge and experience of martial arts, it is only through your practice and understanding that it will become your knowledge.

There is little time spent on technique in this book, but there is much about the context and purpose of training and the fundamentals of practice without which, technique alone will count for little. Within these pages Raymond Towers raises the issue of authenticity within martial arts and life, and the differences between genuine development that encompasses the physical, psychological, emotional and spiritual, and the modern focus of practicing martial arts as little more than 'organised brutality'. Core principles of movement and practice are examined, as well as the strategy and psychology of combat.

Equally importantly Raymond uses this book to address how we can use the martial arts, of whatever style or discipline, to become more authentically ourselves – that is to aim to become our truest and best selves, compassionate, confident, and able to rise to the challenges that face us.

It is in our lives outside the training hall that we are truly put to the test, and while physical confrontation is always a possibility, in reality we are more likely to be required to retain our emotional and psychological balance in the face of much less explosive, but possibly more challenging, situations in our work or relationships. Raymond's book encourages us to see that our progress, both as practitioners of the arts and as people, depends on an ever-deepening understanding of fundamentals, developing solid mental and physical foundations so that we can react spontaneously and effectively.

As a student of Raymond's for some years I have benefited enormously from his teaching, and from practicing the arts. It is a privilege to be asked to write a foreword for a book that I hope will provide insight and inspiration for any student of the martial arts.

Matthew Holtby

Introduction

When an archer is shooting for nothing
He has all his skill.
If he shoots for a brass buckle
He is already nervous
If he shoots for a prize of gold
He goes blind
Or sees two targets
He is out of his mind

His skill has not changed
But the prize divides him
He cares
He thinks more of winning
Than of shooting
And the need to win
Drains him of power.

Anonymous

There is at first sight a strange dichotomy within martial arts philosophy. This dichotomy is to be found in the person who searches and seeks peace and inner serenity while at the same time being engaged in the pursuit of excellence in a fighting art. How do we bring together these two contradictory paths?

What is to be gained from a martial artist stating openly that they strive after peace and tranquility? The origins of martial arts, whether they be the so-called "internal" or "external" systems, stress this doctrine of peace and serenity balanced with an understanding of physical power.

It is true that many martial artists practice some form of meditation, whether it be standing or sitting meditation, focusing on breathing and relaxation. All of these arts emphasise inner peace and tranquility.

Whatever the merits of the thousands of different systems, 'master hands' have always pointed out that perfection of technique must invariably bring with it another step on the road towards perfection of the self. This development of self requires a depth of spirituality, which overcomes the dichotomy mentioned earlier.

It is my belief that it is the responsibility of senior teachers to pass on this knowledge of a spiritual dimension. It is not simply about teaching the effectiveness of a technique, or about providing students with the confidence to walk down increasingly dangerous paths in life.

It is about providing the opportunity to develop and discipline our own characters so that we become not simply strong and effective exponents of a technique, but mature and valued members of society. In this way, rather than acceding to the criteria of others, we become more aware of the serenity, poise and power that resides within us all.

The pursuit of peace and serenity in our studies does not come easily. It requires a discipline and training even more profound than the developing of the physical skills of martial arts. We must allow the complete, full and mature development not only of our physical martial art skills, but also the skills required to be a responsible and mature human being who deals with their feelings appropriately and truthfully.

Without discipline and spirituality the study of martial arts becomes reducible to the extremities of primordial aggression. True understanding comes from discipline; through discipline we attain spirituality, which is so vital to us all. Through an understanding of the spirituality of our study we lift the arts above their potential baseness and imbibe them with sincerity and truthfulness.

In this context the development of peace and serenity must be a central factor in the development of our personal character. The gaining of expertise or ever more ' grades' is of no importance, and ultimately meaningless, if there is no hand in hand gaining of inner peace.

All of us search for an experience of 'something' in our life, that indefinable, ineffable something beyond ourselves that makes sense of our existence and brings order to the chaos of our lives. It is the experience of this something that can redefine the martial arts not simply as fighting systems, but as a legitimate philosophical outlook on life. Thus, what was originally a doctrine of seemingly unresolved tensions can become a method and tool to greater and deeper human development.

This short treatise was never intended, but became an opportunity for me to pass on that 'something' I had the honour of learning from my teachers, and from the classics, but most of all from my own experience of life. This is no New Age treatise; it comes out of many hard knocks both physically and emotionally and is grounded in strong foundations.

Many martial artists spend their lives studying and developing an efficient and effective fighting system. Others will place their emphasis on health and well-being. Yet others will use the arts as a tool to develop their knowledge of their true selves. My journey has passed all these staging posts, from Earth to Me and then to Heaven. Martial Arts that do not encompass the whole lead to frustration, where we continue to live in fear, always reflecting the dialectic of them and me, me against nature where the ego remains supreme.

In writing the way I have, I have followed a traditional pattern and format based upon Eastern Martial and Spiritual Philosophies. I am, however, a Western man, and the interaction between the East and West, between man and woman, not to mention between homo sapiens and nature, is intricate, complex and extremely vulnerable, and should therefore be approached with sensitivity. I hope I have done so in the knowledge of the base from which I have begun.

I hope to offer some guidance, for I believe that the ancient wisdom of the martial arts can be used as a datum point around which men and women can gather, a place where they can gain insight, wisdom and strength with which to face the struggles, challenges and uncertainties which are part of our modern existence. True authenticity understands the wisdom of 'investing in loss', the strength in 'yielding', the 'necessity' of following our true path, our mission, and our lives.

We come to understand the extent to which we must go with the natural forces, which inevitably guide our lives, each piece of knowledge, each step, becoming its own reward.

As warriors, we must learn to give up on the foolish and eventually fruitless objectives in our own training, where we believe our ego will overcome so many self-generated obstacles. Once we have done this we will find that nature travels the same path as ourselves, there are no obstacles to overcome and we are indeed one and the same with the Tao.

Perhaps you have experienced moments when you and your surroundings become one, when it feels so perfect, when you feel right in your time and place, so right that you cannot imagine yourself in a more perfect or harmonious place. At such moments one is experiencing what I have chosen to call true authenticity, the true self; yielding is complete, the ego is quieted, the monkey mind still, the order and wisdom of nature is a given. One stands humbly upon the path, feeling if only for an instant the peace of not seeking, and the gentle embrace of health and wholeness.

The Martial Arts path is a tool for breaking away from our love affair with our egos, a tool that can help prevent over-indulgence in our own appetites. Here we find 'No Fear'. The arts have nudged me in that direction, in the direction of liberation through successive moments of authenticity. The arts can give us a philosophy of clarification, a confirmation of what the authentic self is, what we can be. We can learn again what we have always known, that there is no escaping abusing our body-mind relationship, for nature is with us every step of the way, always moving us and giving us the ability, the chance to change direction.

The immediacy of change is always with us as individuals, and collectively as part of the world community. In order to respond to this change we must be open, flexible and wise, if we are to fulfill our given purpose in life.

I hope these reflective writings will be an inspiration as well as give some pleasure. I hope the written words have the strength to leave the page and become true body-mind actions. Moving us onwards, childlike, to an honest and fully aware meeting with our own true selves in nature, enjoying the journey in the same way that the stream enjoys its own journey back to its source.

Enjoy!

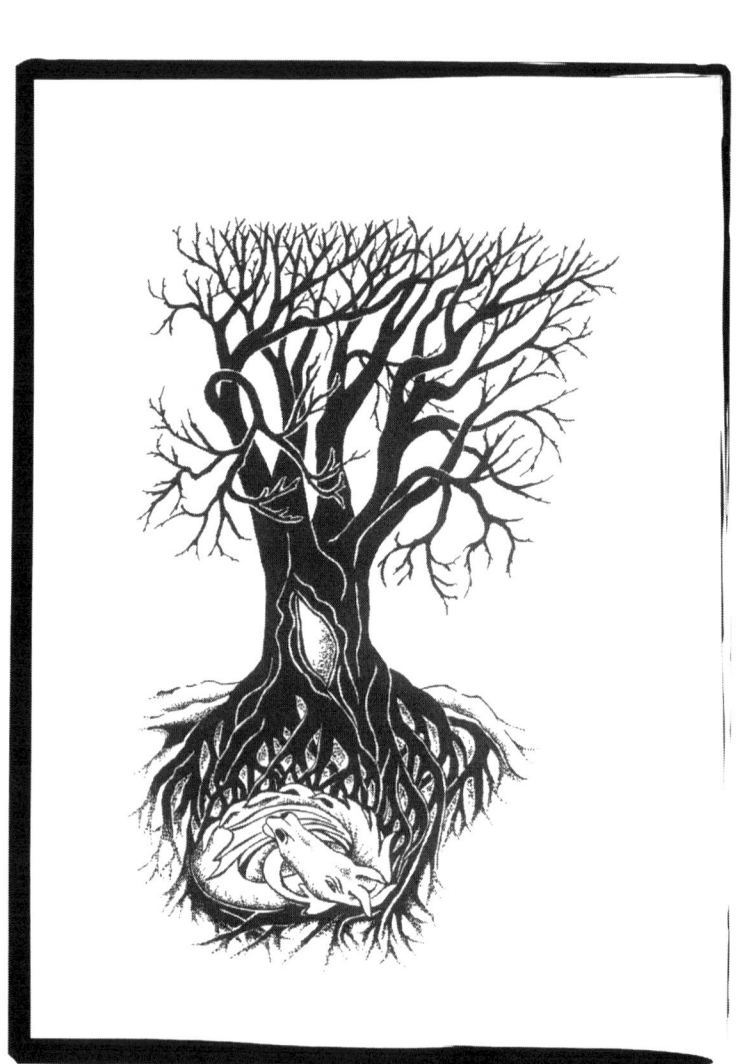

Week One

The goal in Martial Arts practice
is the development of the higher mind,
that is the mind that is active and creative
in harmony with the truth of nature, a symbiotic
coming together of the known and the knower.

This symbiotic coming together demands great
discipline, discipline in this sense means knowing
what you truly want, and the willingness to do whatever
it takes to achieve it.

The starting point is the void, for it is
in the void that you will find your true self in relation to nature.

The natural state is that state where the body, mind,
and spirits are harmoniously unified. From a belief in emptiness
comes calm, from calm comes stillness, the stillness which allows your inner
voice to guide you,
from here the natural state can be realised.

Week Two

Discipline requires a method,
without a method there is no discipline.
The outside and the inside should be as one,
in harmony with life's force.
Your vital energy and that of the universe are one,
there is no separation.
Heaven, earth and you are one;
work for the good by being one with all.

Your practice should develop a high state of awareness
in relation to your life force.
A Martial Artist should walk through life
in harmony with nature,
in such a way that no footprints are left behind.
Masters of the arts take part in life's daily tasks unrecognised,
not because they are secretive,
but because they are living in harmony with nature.

Week Three

Internal Methods

Develop the breath, move the qi.
Harmonise inside and outside.
Become one with your movement;
rise, fall, extend and contract.
Stand above; extend beyond, your consciousness.
Develop yin and yang and understand their meeting point.
Become an empty vessel,
understand that within emptiness you find others weakness.

External Methods

Practice the movements:
advance and withdraw,
empty and full,
moving and bridging.
Use the seven stars to their full:
utilise the external and internal harmonies,
incline neither left or right back or forward.
Use stance, posture and technique appropriately.

Week Four

In the beginning your practice
will be obvious.
With study, patience and perseverance
you will find your own harmony
with the movement
of your particular method, until
it is true and natural.

Do not limit your study of the Martial Arts
to time objectives.
You will learn to understand that
you are a unique individual
and that your practice is dependent on
your own experiences with life.

There is no need or desire to compete
to get to a point before someone else.
Simply practice what you are doing
and you will find your own personal way
to your original source.

Restrain and conceal your skills;
they are not found lightly
and should not be used lightly.
Use your skills and knowledge
with understanding and compassion.

Week Five

The Harmonies

External Harmonies

Shoulders harmonise with the hips.
Elbows harmonise with the knees.
Wrists harmonise with the ankles.

Internal Harmonies

The body harmonises with the mind.
The mind harmonises with the intent.
The intent harmonises with the qi.
The qi harmonises with the spirit.
The spirit harmonises with movement.
The movement harmonises with emptiness.

Functional Harmonies

Neck, spine and lower back.
Shoulders, elbows, wrists and hands.
Hips, knees, ankles and feet.
Mind, eyes and seven stars.

Week Six

Your practice begins with development
of your strength and flexibility.
Work from the inside out;
do not fall into the trap of seeing this development
only in the physical realm.

Learn well not to be there:
your opponent strikes, you are not there,
they grasp you, there is nothing to hold.
If you are there and you need to respond,
respond only with the energy necessary,
do not waste your own life force.

Appear empty whilst being full;
you can only develop this state by being quiet,
by knowing yourself.
Your art should be seamless, natural.

You should learn to receive and express without form.
You take your life's adversary's balance by being balanced,
you neutralise life's attacks by being neutral;
these are the necessary components of your development.

Week Seven

Develop the virtues of discrimination, tolerance, forgiveness, contentment, detachment and humility.

Beware the five passions of lust, anger, greed, attachment and vanity.

Learn meditative techniques that develop calmness. Constantly return to these techniques delving ever deeper with time, until your calm is natural in the context of your own nature.

Through calmness you will maintain your centre, rooted inside and outside, balanced. Through being centred and balanced your intention is unknown; if your intentions are obvious then you will be lost.

Practice in order to gain knowledge and understanding. The more you advance on your own development, the more practice is needed. Joy comes from practice, in this joy you will find your own true nature.

Week Eight

Regulate the breath, ensure you are in control of your breath
at all times, not your breath in
control of you. Once you reach a point where you lose
control of the breath you lose your
physical and mental balance.

The breath should be calm, quiet and smooth to enable the flow of
life's energy, qi, for it is the
smooth and regulated flow of qi, which will define your actions.

In a situation of conflict you are responsible for your actions. The
diligence of your practice will
be expressed through your response.
What you do today, will become tomorrow's condition.

Always return to balance; the recovery rate of any athlete is of
prime importance. It is your
responsibility as a martial artist to regain balance in your
environment as soon as possible, so that
harmony can once more be restored.

Week Nine

Rules of Engagement

For the higher state the first rule of engagement with your adversaries is not
to
be there.
If the first rule is compromised then the second rule is not
to be unbalanced,
you stay balanced through a state of no action.

If the second rule is compromised, then the third rule is to
take decisive action
returning to a state of harmony swiftly.

There is a time and place for everything.
Be always sensitive to this adage.
Remain open and accepting
so that you can receive any energy, hard or soft,
and then respond appropriately.

Always remain quiet and calm;
through the practice of standing you can become fearless
and thereby control your environment.
You decide when and how you deal with aggression;
soft or hard they are of equal stature
if developed from a position of balance.

Week Ten

The Dilemma of Contradictions

There is no future, there is no past,
only now, this is where your focus is in all situations.

Step forward decisively with the front foot,
step back with the rear,
be equal in the clarity of movement
and take advantage of the half step.

Step backwards in a straight line with a curved step.
Turn the body in with the toe-in step;
always move from the centre of your heart
and the centre of your body.

When going forward
always enter through your adversary's middle door.

Strengthen the bow,
and fire the arrow of intent straight;
practice in curves, but when taking action
use the effectiveness of the straight line.

When attacked, evade.
When it is to your advantage, yield;
redirect the negative energy and place it in the void
where the strength dissipates.

Week Eleven

The Strategies

Remember that any offensive strategy is flawed from the outset
for it is borne out of mental and physical insecurity and imbalance.

Use stillness whilst in motion,
using movement to deal with change,
use the tip and move the root,
use the whole force to ensure a correct motion.

Be aware of the ten directions;
be alert and nimble,
always being ready to accept change,
for attachment creates stagnation.

Always be ready to change places with your aggressor,
using strategy to control clumsiness.

Use slanting to return to straight,
straight to deal with slanting,
solid to deal with empty,
and empty to deal with solid.

Be sensitive to the forms of the monkey's head,
the snake's eyes, the turtle's back,
the dragon's waist, the chicken's walk and tiger's step;
all are important and should mould into one.

Week Twelve

Make the difference between double and single weightedness clear;
single weighted will always give you the advantage.

Lead your adversary into an empty house,
the emptier you become, the closer to nature and fuller you become.

One natural truth is that change is constant;
understand this and you will truly begin to understand your arts.

Store the power of the Earth in you legs,
ensure all the joints are curved and flexible,
allow the major energy gates of the body to become connected.

Round the back with the shell of a turtle,
round the arms, embrace the tree,
open the energy gate of the kidneys,
express the energy through your techniques,
thereby transforming all that you do in relationship to life's force.

Learn to lock away the monkey mind, so you can be clear about
your true intentions.
Let your eyes shine bright with your true self; clear away the
noise that surrounds us all.

Week Thirteen

At all times reserve the greater part of your energy for yourself,
so when necessary you can give to others.

Hold in your dreams;
remember, the eye of the tiger never loses its intent.
Beware of grace;
the tiger's steps are a living expression of such grace.

The five hearts and the six harmonies work together
to create a whole in tune with nature.

Wait calmly, so that when conflict raises itself it will
already have been dealt with.

Calmness, balance, harmony are developed through practice,
perseverance and patience.

Closed-door teaching is yours alone,
there are no secrets, there are only stages in learning.

Move like a River and stand like a Mountain;
the river flows to its source, the mountain soars to its peak,
the journey is long in both directions,
but your perseverance will see you through.

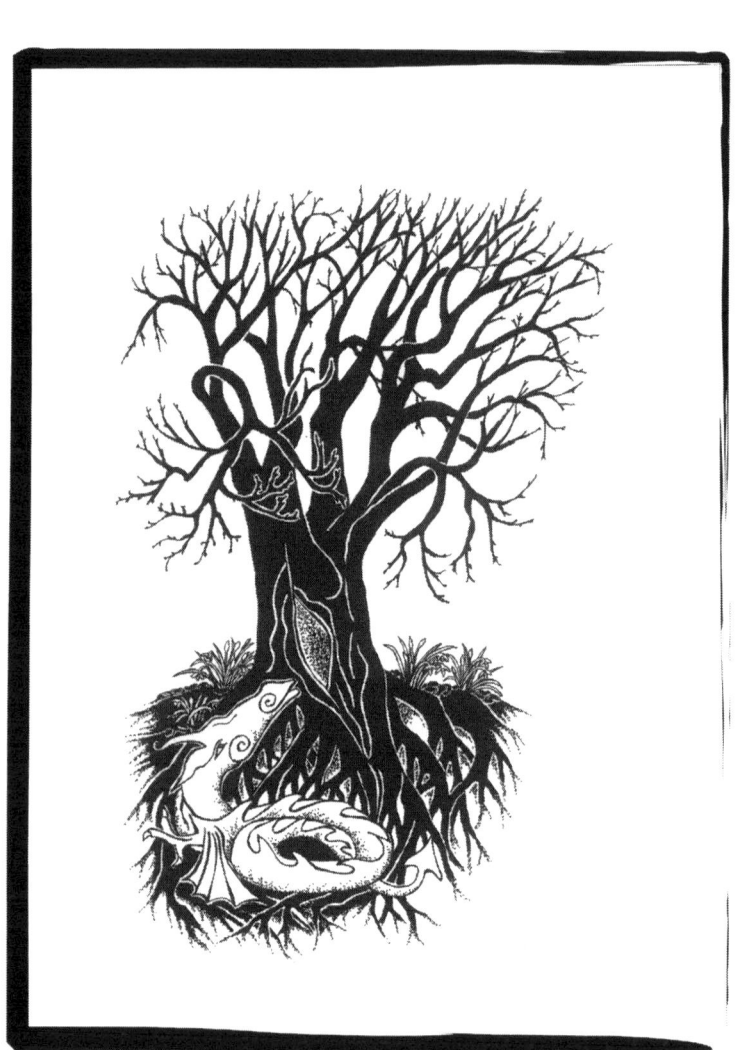

Week Fourteen

Remember that before one can build a great temple
you must build firm foundations;
the basics are the advanced regardless of which art you practice.

The most advanced skills come through the direct experience
of that which you practice.

Any worthwhile endeavour takes self-discipline and determination,
there is no progress without practice, and you always have the choice.
In your perseverance be sure to recognise wisdom
and intelligently balance your relationship to nature.

Remember your ambassadorial role in the interaction with society;
honour and respect those who have gone before you.

Be a positive example to all you meet;
let yours be a moral and ethical approach that can be recognised by anyone,
let gratitude and service be your natural self.
Do not allow these to be empty words.

The one moves the whole,
the whole moves the one;
there is no separation.

Week Fifteen

Do not overtax the Yi (mind) because this will weaken the bones,
this in turn weakens the vital energy of the kidneys,
turning strength into weakness.

Maintain the circles in the external harmonies,
the functional harmonies and the five hearts.

Let your energy rise from the Earth through the feet to the hands
and finally to the top of the head.
Let it then rise and envelop your immediate surroundings.

The Trinity of Earth, You and Heaven then become one.

Use expansion and contraction in equal measure to gather your power.

When you are still, then the internal system begins its circling;
like an eddying stream let your life force fill every nook and cranny
with the joy and light of nature itself.

Through opening and closing you adapt to any and
all conditions and changes.

Week Sixteen

Where the mind goes the qi follows.
Be careful then why, where and how you place your intention.

It is important to know that technique is not superior to posture,
that posture is not superior to stance,
for technique can only express the strength
of the posture and stance.

Ensure that your technique is light and fluid,
controlled by the spine and your spirit.

Your joints are the energy sluice gates for your body,
connecting the joints transfers and transforms
your energy throughout the system.

Knowing this then take care to daily mobilise your joints;
when you exercise your joints and ligaments together
your body becomes physically connected.

Strengthen your blood, breath and bones for greater health.
A warrior must be healthy as well as fit,
full of life's energy to embrace the daily challenges that face us all.

Week Seventeen.

Keep the golden elixir – saliva – always clean and full in your mouth,
for it is the first line of self-defence. Use this knowledge.

Kan, the fire energy, and Li, the water essence, must be in balance.
Keep your head cool and your feet warm.

The beginning is the end, the end is the beginning,
as it is in life, then it is in your study of the arts.
This is important.

Develop your physical, then your health.
On this foundation you will build your spiritual life.
Be mentally agile;
never depend on physical strength or martial technique.

Week Eighteen

Your practice begins and ends
with respect;
respect for yourself and for others.

Without respect for our true nature
our practice degenerates into no more than
organised abuse.

Abuse of nature, of others,
is not the way
of the arts.

Ritual is often seen by some
as a substitute for respect.
There is no substitute for respect;
it must come form the heart.

Week Nineteen

'There is no greater martial art':
in the same way as there is no greater lifestyle.
This is an illusion tied to our egos.
The martial art is dependent on the practitioner.

Defining the qualities of one's art
is not tied to technique, tricks or strategies
for overcoming, for winning.

You must define the quality of your art
through the quality of your life, for
all the arts must be controlled by the mind and spirit.

Development is growing in awareness,
awareness of our own strengths and weaknesses,
this is where our training should focus.

Only with this awareness
can we develop our strategy,
not for combat,
but for life.

Week Twenty

Do not chain your mind
like a dog chained to a post,
let it roam freely.

Do not then be chained to a master
or to a system,
for then you are chained to a post of
your own making.

The beginner lives in fear
of opening their minds,
in fear of allowing it to roam free;
without a free mind you can never reach
your full potential.

Week Twenty-One

The higher martial mind
goes beyond your practice of the arts;
it must inform everything that we do in our lives.

Always be aware of your actions;
be diligent in your method,
use those methods that
are in harmony with nature.

Only in this way will the spirit grow
as one with our own nature.

True development is a life-time endeavour,
competence in the techniques
is not true development.

Having no desire for martial success,
no need for pride,
no necessity to humble oneself;
this is true evolution.

Week Twenty-Two

Develop by becoming a better human being
not a better martial artist;
be better now than you were, be better in the future
than you are.

Remember:
whatever you do, your spiritual life is at stake;
do not take this lightly.
Whether you are immersed in the culture of the East or West
nature does not discriminate.

You prepare for life, for the arts,
in one way; the way of being true to yourself.
This is why understanding oneself is so important.

Week Twenty-Three

Through correct breathing we adjust and balance our body,
giving us the ability to perform actions efficiently.
Whilst inhaling we prepare the body,
whilst exhaling the body executes the movement.
Without the correct balance of adjustment and movement
the body becomes inefficient.

The basic movements of breathing
are up and down, in and out,
expand and contract.

Breathing is like the wind;
it prevents stagnation
which in its turn
ensures good health.

There are three stages of breathing;
Natural, Deep, Natural.
Understand these stages
and you will understand life.

Week Twenty-Four

An understanding of the sections in alignment with breath
is necessary to become a competent warrior.

The legs have their root in the hips,
their middle in the knees,
their tips in the feet.

The torso has its root in the abdomen,
its middle in the chest,
its tip on the head.

The arms have their root in the shoulders
their middle in the elbows,
their tip in the hands.

The legs are the root,
the torso the middle,
the arms the tips.

Utilise your breath,
breathing efficiently into your tips,
unifying the whole body.

Week Twenty-Five

Every movement should have intent.
Every posture should have intent.
Intent guides the practice
from beginning to end.

Each strike must be preceded by intent;
do not make your intent visible.
Then it is possible to move,
turn and move, move together,
stick, connect and follow,
jump and dodge,
turn over and leave empty,
ward off and roll back,
push and press down.

Do not strike with the fist beyond five feet.
Beyond three feet do not use the elbows.
Close in do not use the hands.
Use one step, one strike.

Week Twenty-Six

Attacking when your opponent is prepared is foolish.
Striking where your opponent has intention is foolish.

Take advantage of all attacks,
soft and full, empty and solid;
evade solid and attack empty.

If attacked by many, show no fear.
Respond as if there is only one;
attack the one.

You must be able to move
back, forward, to all angles
soft and hard.

Be like a Mountain,
watch like an Eagle,
always ready to take the advantage.

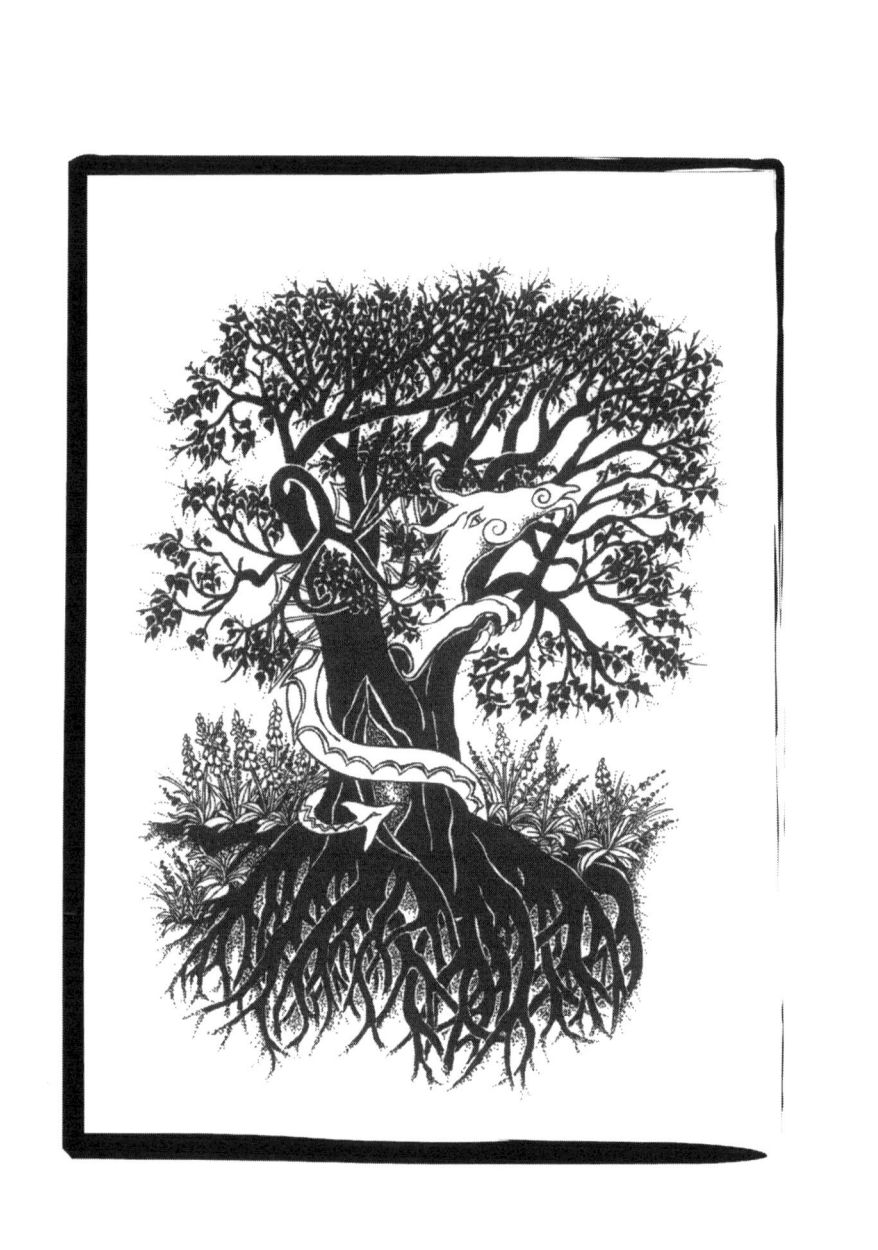

Week Twenty-Seven

Always act decisively.
Aim for your opponent's middle line.
The whole of your body must be as one.

Dodging is advancing, advancing is dodging.
Striking is protecting, protecting is striking.

When attacking left, enter at the right.
When attacking right, enter at the left.

Let the heel be the first to touch the ground.
Let the seven stars be fully empowered.

The Yi is all.
The body, the bowstring.
The hands are like arrows.

Week Twenty-Eight

The five rules of development

First rule:
Progress must be gradual.

Second rule:
The arts should prolong life,
not make it shorter.

Third Rule:
Perseverance:
The time is worth the effort.

Fourth Rule:
Develop a quiet mind,
leave ego to others.

Fifth Rule:
Observe and understand the past,
showing respect at all times.

Week Twenty-Nine

The heart,
the eyes,
the hands.

Correct martial application
is the same as correct living:
invisible.

Look to the front of the face,
look to the front of the torso,
look beyond the feet.

Week Thirty

Neglect the basic skills at your peril;
stances, postures and techniques
are the basic skills.

Your practice is the practice
of basic skills.
All should be related to your
unified body movement.

The unified body is the
center of you.
You become firm, you become rooted.
You become the natural you.

Week Thirty-One

Beware of holding the breath,
for this can damage the lungs,
stopping the freedom
of flow.

Beware of holding your strength in any particular part of the
body to exert force,
for this can cause blood stagnation in that part.

Beware of pushing out the chest
or sucking in the abdomen,
for all of these will deplete the efficiency
of the lungs, thereby blocking of energy.

These are natural laws which should be followed
diligently.

The sleeping dragon is awakened by thunder.
Strong winds bend the limbs of even great trees.
Take precautions internally by keeping stable internally.

Week Thirty-Two

When you are rooted and balanced,
your actions will be strong.
An action without root and balance
will not be successful,
even executed a thousand times.

When your yi is agile
your actions will be clear and efficient;
your intentions will be invisible
but your actions will be known to all.

When you can apply Yin and Yang together
you will be able to channel your power
into soft and hard whenever you wish.
This is great accomplishment.

Week Thirty-Three

When martial artists neglect the cultivation
of their inner life
they become machines,
slaves to the materialism of form.
In this case they are martial artists in name only.

Week Thirty- Four

He meditates when walking,
he meditates when sitting.
Silent, speaking, resting,
his body is at peace.
In the face of pointed swords
he remains calm.

Week Thirty-Five

The Five restrictions state:

Do not be frivolous.

Do not be conceited.

Do not be impatient.

Do not be negligent.

Do not be lascivious.

The Seven Detriments State:

Fornication depletes the energy,

Anger harms the breath,

Worry numbs the mind,

Over trustfulness hurts the heart,

Too much alcohol dilutes the blood,

Laziness softens the muscles,

Tenseness weakens the bones.

Without discipline, laziness controls your life.

Week Thirty-Six

Understand the art of breathing,
nourish the chi.

Those who know the art of breathing
have the strength, wisdom and courage of ten tigers.
Serious contemplation cannot be rushed.
Where there is no evil, there is no disruption.
Purify the thoughts by listening to your breathing,
just the sounds of inhaling and exhaling;
this brings internal purification,
this brings life.

Week Thirty-Seven

The warrior's path is a life long study;
it is a serious investment.
An attitude of calm endurance and self-possession
must be acquired,
persist in what you have begun.
Those who command patience may command
what they will.
Talent grows strong through personal force,
character becomes firm through
the Yi.

Week Thirty-Eight

Do not be trapped by technique,
do not be direct in your defence or attack.
Your movements remain unseen, elusive and circular
like your life is circular.
Harmonise the body and mind
so they move as one;
there is no deadlier weapon than the will,
the sharpest sword is not equal to it.
Through the pursuit of unity in action
you will conquer all before you.

Week Thirty-Nine

The warrior seeks no advantage,
makes no plans,
engages in no business.
The Tao is all they seek.

At one with nature they remain soft like water,
gaining poise and power,
through patient understanding
of change.

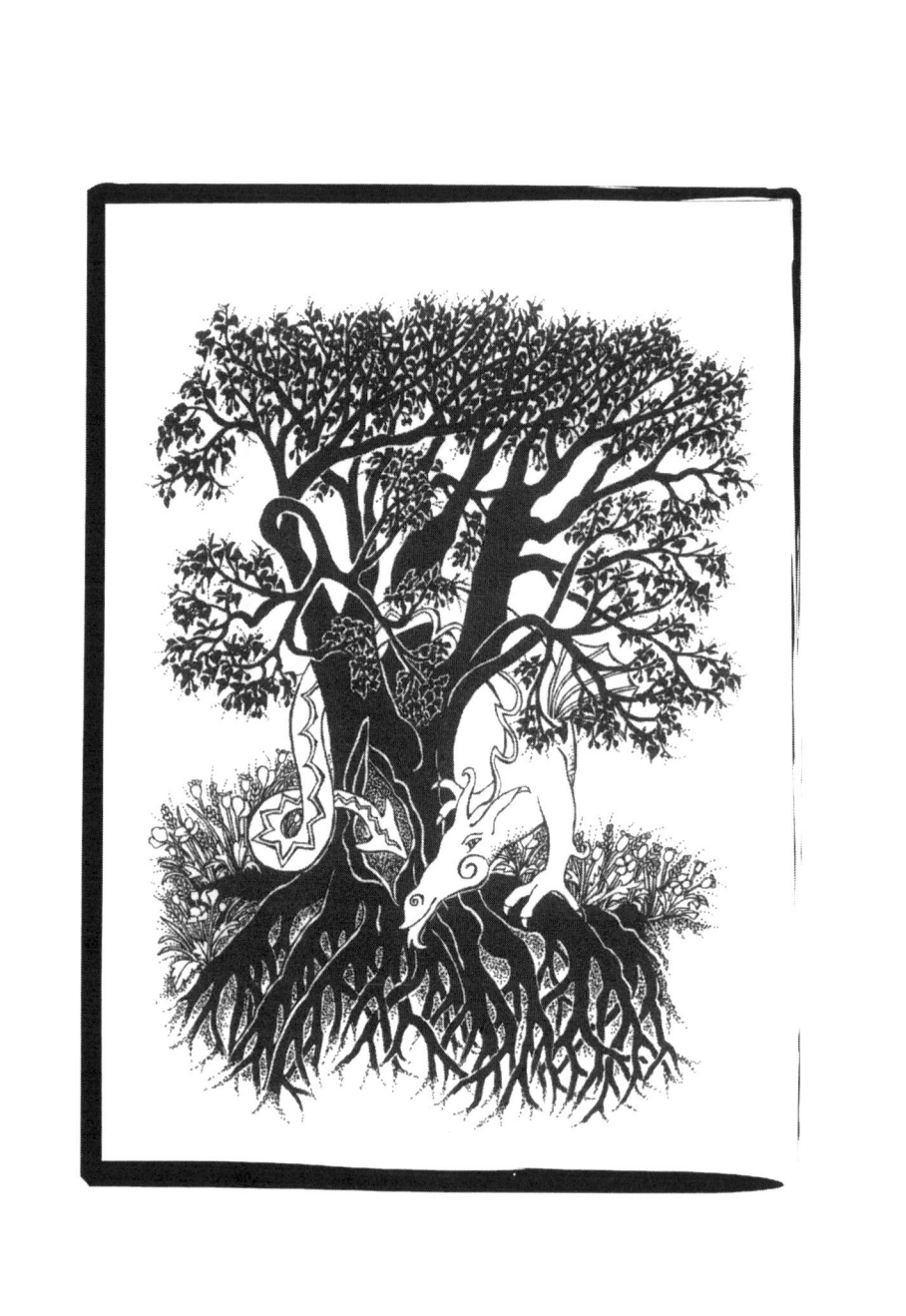

Week Forty

To be a warrior you must be true
to yourself.
It is something you must want to do,
it is not a game for the faint hearted.
It is an acquired discipline,
a character-building path, which lasts
a lifetime.

Do not waste your time.
Do not waste your life.
If you choose the discipline then dedicate
yourself to its study,
listen to your teachers, watch and learn,
but listen to yourself;
use your time wisely for it is indeed
precious.

Week Forty-One

A hidden strength resides in us all.
This supernormal power is developed
through the exercise of a firm resolve.

In the midst of violence the warrior
shows total determination,
thereby determining the outcome.

Lax actions will only create an advantage
for the opponent,
therefore development of willpower,
perseverance of the mind, is paramount in
ensuring the physical body can overcome an attack.

Week Forty-Two

Mental turmoil slows down reflexes;
the calm mind is necessary
for the efficient application of technique.

The greatest safety is in the
eye of the hurricane,
the warrior's mind remains detached.

The conquest of mental turmoil,
the monkey mind,
leads to a peaceful existence.

Week Forty-Three

Avoid unnecessary movement;
through the conservation of energy
the warrior will keep their body
stronger for longer.

Intuitive and decisive response to an outside force
produces maximum effect with minimum effort.
This takes time and experience,
but is the goal of your practice.

Human Energy,
after repeated transmission of power,
diminishes,
then becomes ineffective.

Week Forty-Four

Balance:
total and effective power
comes through balance.
The warrior's goal is to retain balance
at all times.

It is not the warrior's objective to take another's balance,
it is the warrior's objective to retain his own balance.
Practice the art of balance at all times,
for it is the key to life.

Week Forty-Five

Always take the shortest and most direct route,
taking control with the least effort.

Do not over extend your body,
for this leads to loss of efficiency,
loss of whole body force.

Get there first with the most
by using the least.

Make your movements, when necessary, conclusive.

Week Forty-Six

To understand humanity is to understand
yourself and all others;
condemnation of the faults of others
show your own faults.

Confucius said that if you respect others
they will respect you.
If you have sympathy for others
they will have sympathy for you.

Seek the wisdom, goodness, and beauty in others
so that you may honour them everywhere.

Week Forty-Seven

Man: the chi circulates.
The chi goes from shoulders to fingers,
the chi goes from thigh to the foot,
the chi goes from vertebrae
to the top of the head.

Earth: the chi penetrates.
Chi goes to the tantien,
chi focuses on the sole,
chi permeates the entire body.

Heaven: Interpreting energy.
'Heat' energy,
understand energy,
the summit.

Week Forty-Eight

In the beginning
your understanding is limited,
you know something
but what you know is not
complete or correct.

Then you build a strong foundation
in your stances, postures and techniques.

You now excel, you have internalised yourself,
your movements;
you create your own style.

Your skills are now consummated,
you know yourself.

Week Forty-Nine

To save energy,
to accumulate energy,
to increase the power of energy:
these are prerequisite if we wish
to use energy.

Those who have found life's energy,
the strong, calm, invincible life,
these warriors place themselves where
there are no boundaries.

Striving no more to become,
they are all that
they have longed for.

All about them is life,
within them is life,
before them is life.

Week Fifty

To be a true warrior
is to find the limitless possibilities
that reside within us all.

To make this discovery
is to know that we may undertake anything
and never fail.

We can be all that we can be when we learn to use
what nature has already implanted firmly within us:
to be still and to live.

Week Fifty-One

In each movement
body and spirit must be united.

The way of the warrior
is dependent
on spirit.

Only when there is sufficient spirit
can the techniques
be complete.

The warrior strives to conserve
Essence,
hold on to energy,
guard their spirit.

Integrate with nature,
learning to respond to the wind
of change calmly.

Week Fifty-Two

Warriors develop
harmony,
inside and outside,
posture that makes
the energy smooth.

Be alert,
or one becomes rigid.

Guide all actions from
the mind.

When quiet, as stable
as a mountain.

When in action as powerful
as wind and thunder.

Have Eight methods on the hands,
Five directions under the feet.

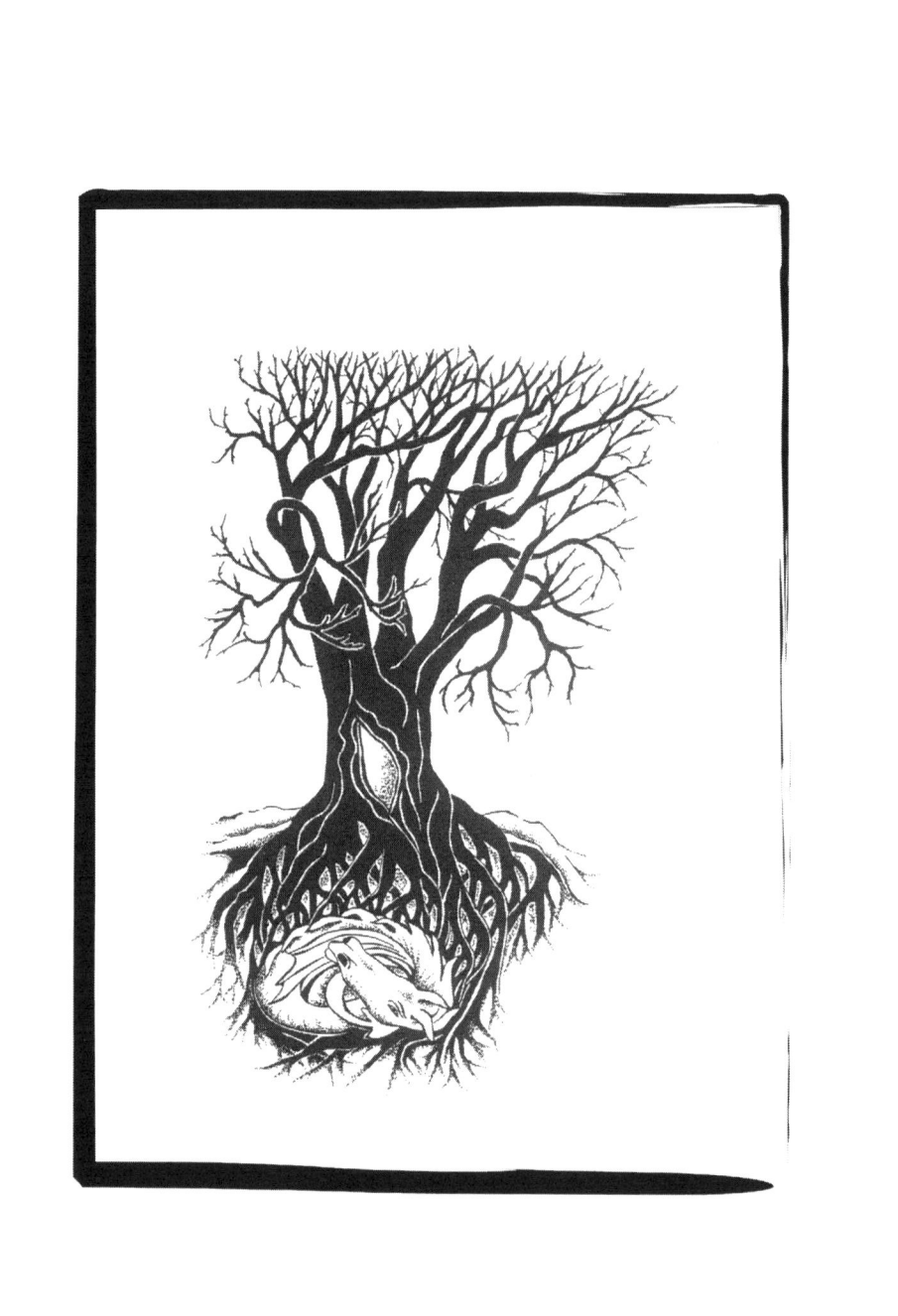

If a warrior understands the theory, if they persevere, are
patient and true to
themselves, then they can reach the highest of states where
the mind can roam
freely in accord with nature. Then they can be in control of their
own destiny,
full of life, full of joy and full of love.

Raymond Towers

Postscript

I have included this Postscript in order to give the reader a flavour of the source of my own thoughts, which have been the basis for this book.

Martial Arts have always been an integral part of human existence; these arts contain valuable lessons that can prepare us in coping with all the challenges life can place in all our paths. For me the Arts continue to serve both as a means of self-defence and as a way to discipline my mind, body and spirit. Through the understanding of our mind and body we learn about ourselves, through understanding ourselves we can begin the process of living in harmony with our environment.

True attainment in the Arts is internal, it is not visible to others, but others can feel it in the way we interact with all those around us. What I have attempted to do in the pages that have preceded this postscript is pass on the knowledge I have gained in just thirty-five years of study. However as a teacher I have come to learn that a teacher cannot make the student learn, nor can they just give away their knowledge and ability to the student. The student has the responsibility to train and assimilate the knowledge and ability by themselves. A teacher has to be willing to teach and the student willing to learn in order for knowledge to flow freely and effectively, so that they can cultivate the Dao together. The songs below are examples from the Internal Arts of Taijiquan, Xingyiquan and Baguazhang which were written by masters of the past with the objective of guiding our cultivation, given freely, their knowledge is indeed worth its weight in gold, studied diligently it can open all doors.

Xingyiquan Classics

Xingyiquan has only a limited number of routines or forms, these reflect the art's principles. Whilst from a point of view of how much there is to learn it can be said to be easy, it can be difficult to understand the deeper essence and meaning of the art. Xingyiquan is an internal art which nourishes qi. It follows Qigong theory and principles which include converting essence into qi, using the qi to nourish the spirit, purifying the qi and attaining the Dao.

The Song of Fighting

The Body

In the technique of striking, you must move your body first.
It is real only when your hands and feet arrive together.
The fist is shaped like a cannon, the body like a dragon,
when encountering the opponent.
Your body becomes as if on fire.

When striking the Yi is generated, the head is the centre.
When the entire body arrives together, the opponent cannot defend.
The feet step in the centre door,
occupying the advantage.
If your opponent is not skilled,
he will be taken.

The Shoulder

When the shoulder is striking for one Yin,
you return with one yang.
Keeping both hands hidden in dark places.
Left and right strikes.
The power depends upon the posture.

The Hand

When the hands strike Yi is on the opponent's chest.
You are a tiger leaping towards the lamb.
When you stick firmly and use Li,
they should be extended and loose.
The elbows hidden under the armpits.

When moving forward, left or right,
firmly with jian jin.
When the hands move at the mind's command,
the opponent will be beaten easily.

When the fist are used for striking,
the shape of the three sections cannot be seen.
If the shape and the shadows can be seen,
then the strike is not good.
Proficiency in the strike comes at the end of the thought
and does not dally with the thought.
It is generated before and not after the qi.

The Hips

When the hips are striking.
left and right should be relaxed
moving easily.
The exchange of both feet natural.

When the hips are used for striking the middle section
both hips should be connected.
Yin and Yang combined is difficult to obtain.
If the hips are like fish on dry land,
your intentions will be easily seen.

When the hips and the tail
are used for striking,
movement up and down are hidden,
it is fierce like a tiger
leaving its cave.

The Knees

When using the knees for striking they are deadly.
Two hands feint movement in the upper centre.
This is something you must practice with diligence.
Unlimited happiness can be gained.

When the knees are used for striking,
many places can be hit.
Without your opponent's knowledge.
The knees should strike like a tiger
breaking from its cage.

The body turning smoothly,
your movements strong and efficient.
Repel left and right clearly.
Strike as desired.

The Feet

When the feet step, the Yi must be firm and accurate.
Not entering emptiness.
The key is in the rear legs springing forward action.
When storing your Yi, do not let your opponent
sense your movement.
When you move it should be like a tornado.

Taijiquan

Over the last few centuries many songs and poems have been written about Taijiquan. These words have played an essential role in preserving the knowledge and wisdom of past masters of the arts, although in many cases the identity of the authors and the dates of origin have been lost. Below are words attributed to Wang Zong Yu, a renowned master of Taijiquan who is believed to have lived from 1736-1796.

Taiji in Taijiquan

Wang Zong-Yu said
'What is Taiji'?
It is generated from Wuji
It is a pivotal function
of movement and stillness.
It is the mother of Yin and Yang.

When it moves it divides,
at rest it unites.
From this we know that Taiji
is not Wuji, nor is it yin and yang.

This natural pivotal function of
movement and stillness
is named Dao.

When Yin and Yang are divided
the two polarities are established.
From the two is generated the four phases,
from the four phases comes Bagua.
From the Bagua comes the sixty four trigrams,
from the sixty four comes all.

In the practice of Taijiquan
Yin and Yang must be understood.
To know Yin and Yang
you must know Taiji.
To know Taiji then you need
to comprehend the Dao

Before movement in Taijiquan
Xin should be peaceful,
Qi harmonious.
Xin and Yi are at the Dantien,
Qi stays in its residence.

On reaching the state of calmness
you are in Wuji.
When Xin and Yi act the qi begins to circulate,
the body moves and the Yin and Yang divide.

Xin and Yi are what is called Taiji in Taijiquan.
The Dao of Taijiquan
is the Dao of Xin and Yi

We are between Heaven and Earth,
Xin and Yi have unlimited scope,
neither restricted by time or space.
From Xin and Yi
we initiate Yin and Yang,
therefore in learning Taijiquan
you must train Xin and Yi.

Xin and Yi are contained internally.
This belongs to Yin,
the movements belong to Yang.
Xin and Yi direct us to the Dao
cultivating our true nature.

It is said that Taijiquan originated
from Daoism.
The ultimate goal of Daoism
is the unification of Heaven and Earth and yourself.
Practicing Taijiquan aids a greater understanding of life.

Baguazhang

This marvellous boxing method, wrote Li Zi Ming in 1982, when practiced correctly according to the essentials, can develop the practitioners physical health to restore the essence, tonify the brain, dispel illness, prolong life and maintain optimum vitality. Li Zi Ming lived until the age of 93, through a period of dynamic and traumatic changes in China's history. The fact that he did live for so long in good health is testament to the benefits he espoused to Baguazhang. Below is a translation of his teacher's Liang Zhen Pu's song on Walking the Circle.

The Song of Circle Walking

Circle Walking depends upon Yin and Yang,
five elements and six harmonies.
Seven stars and eight steps from nine palaces,
one distinguishes firmness and gentleness
internally and externally in all three levels.

All unites into one energy
on a supporting foundation,
four aspects and four angles stabilise eight directions.
The body follows the Ko Bu steps,
releases force in the four tips,
magnify energy by walking and turning.

The forward palm extends like an ox tongue
in false and true gestures.
The rear hand below the elbow keeps.
Advance in orderly ways and retreat with methods,
change and turn the palm in Yin and Yang.
Oblique seems the front in erect and straight,
transverse and flexion.
Turning and rotation in circling
controlled by waist and hips.

Internally five elements are expressed in the tips,
externally five elements are distinguished
through observation.
Internally the Qi travels in all three sections,
externally the hand methods are distinguished
in Yin and Yang.

Walking the circle is separated
into eight directions,
in body movement pay attention to intent and Qi.
Be supple in turning and changing,
do not stop to hold postures,
yield infinite power high, low, far and near.

The waist movements coordinate the four tips,
the eyes watch all eight directions.
The hands harmonise with changing situations,
applications change appropriately,
protecting left and right.

The shoulders should harmonise
from Yin to Yang,
the torso harmonises so rotation is strong.
The hips should harmonise in order to
close in on the opponent.

The knees harmonise close to the side
of the opponent's body.
The feet harmonise for rapid retreat and advance.
The strength of the waist and hips
permeate dodging, extending, leaping and shifting.

In the head strike the intent leads the movement,
the force comes from the waist and hips.
When rising and falling maintain central equilibrium.
The feet bring you into
the opponent's centre gate, to be in a superior position.

The palm thrusts straight out in piercing palm,
striking quickly high and low.
When the opponent's palm strikes, the lead
hand protects the head.
Whilst the elbow strikes with the
intention of piercing the chest.

The back remains stretched,
the chest remains relaxed,
the grain duct pulled upwards.
The shoulder and hip strike
with Yin and Yang confluence.

Containing the Qi depends upon correct body work,
both hands remain in front of the chest.
Pushing, pressing up, leading and guiding;
all follow the body's force.
Move away, close off, split advancing quickly
high and low.

The Eight Postures and eight fundamental palms
originate from continuous turning,
use palm techniques as a basis for understanding
sword and spear.
If one studies the traditional writings
one can understand the theory of Eight Diagram Palm.

If one applies the theory martially,
one understand the theory of change
and is thereby victorious.
Boxing skills of senior masters
are passed down today,
but very seldom can common people
grasp the truth.

Don't blame the conservative of ancestors,
just regret that we have not practiced enough.
To fathom logic and comprehend the theories,
one realises that if the tree has luxuriant
leaves and branches its roots must go deep.

Eight Diagram Palm skills begin with
walking the circle,
only by thoroughly investigating this method
can one realise its true utility.
Erect the head, drop the shoulders and
flow energy downwards.
Direct Qi to the dantien area
For even out-flow and in-flow.

The arm is divided into three sections
for practical applications,
The body work must be equally expressed in the four tips.
The circle around which one walks
is separated into eight directions,
each represented by a character.

The hand and body move together,
all is filled with vitality.
Contract and lift the anus to hold primordial Qi,
the arms extend like an ape's,
the back broad like a bear's,
the body moves with the power of the tiger,
and the supple grace of a dragon.

When facing an opponent it is advisable
to seek the wrist,
move the hands and find advantage
in the footwork.
Move up, down, back, forth, right and left,
move inside and outside,
strike with the shoulders, elbows, knees and hips.

Extend the thigh without it being seen,
in Eight Diagram Palm, from beginning to end
the thigh is the root.
In thirty-six movements, front, back, right and left,
the foot moves diagonally and raises smoothly
with certainty.
Advance and retreat, hook and lift with obvious
and hidden leg work.

Continuously exchanging Yin and Yang
whilst turning,
stomping thrusting to the side,
kicking straight out with the heel,
whirling, bending, piercing, tripping.
All of these one may use as one pleases
after being trained to perfection.

Even if one is highly skilled,
one must still teach methodically,
this prevents the student from wasting time,
exerting himself for nothing.
While skills are obtained in learning martial arts,
they are developed in proper order
so one skill does not impede
the development of another.

Everyone respects outstanding skill,
when the learning process is at a high level,
one will surpass all others.

Everyone respects outstanding skill,
when the learning process is at a high level,
one will surpass all others.

Printed in Poland
by Amazon Fulfillment
Poland Sp. z o.o., Wrocław